"THE TRUTH ON DIABETES: WHAT THEY DIDN'T TELL YOU"

(by a Naturopathic Doctor)

DR. LUMINITA ALEXE, ND

-Naturopathic Doctor

About the author

Dr. Luminita Alexe, ND
– Naturopathic Doctor / Functional Medicine

Dr. Luminita Alexe is a Functional Medicine Physician practicing in Sherman Oaks, CA. Her clinical focus is Diabetes, and she has successfully reversed Diabetes for thousands of her patients using natural medicine.

Dr. Alexe graduated from the National University of Health Science with a Doctor of Naturopathic Medicine Degree and holds a California medical license.

Previous to medical school, Dr. Alexe obtained her Bachelor of Science in Clinical Nutrition/Dietetics from the Loyola University of Chicago. She is a Doctor and a Clinical Nutritionist.

http://www.drlumi.com

TABLE OF CONTENTS

Introduction *1*

Chapter 1 .... *5*

   The Different Types Of Diabetes *5*

Chapter 2 .... *16*

   The Risks Of Treating Diabetes With Drugs Are FAR Worse Than The Disease *16*

Chapter 3 .... *23*

   Stress And Blood Sugar *23*

Chapter 4 .... *25*

   "Diabesity"; Obesogens, Weight, And Diabetes *25*

Chapter 5 .... *32*

   Diabetes And Your Gut *32*

Chapter 6 .... *38*

   10 Reasons For Blood Sugar Swings *38*

Chapter 7: *42*

   Natural Supplements That INCREASE Your Blood Sugar *42*

Chapter 8 .... *45*

   Diabetic Diet No-No's *45*

Chapter 9 .... *54*

   10 Diabetic Superfoods *54*

Chapter 10 .... *60*

   In The End: You Can Reverse Type 2 Diabetes! *60*

INTRODUCTION

Conventional medicine is miserably failing diabetic patients everywhere. The USA consumes 75% of all the medications produced in the world, yet we are only 4% of the world's population. We consume the bulk of the world's drugs and rank #46 in health and longevity according to the World Health Organization.

According to the American Diabetic Association, the staggering costs of diabetes costs America $322 Billion dollars in drug therapy alone. Despite these astronomical costs, it has not helped diabetics. Every DAY thousands of diabetics will develop blindness, kidney failure, heart failure and gangrene/amputation.

The American people should find this medical care unacceptable. The way our medical model works is that we treat symptoms and not the root of the problem. I'm here to tell you that there are other root causes of diabetes and once you find a physician willing to dig a little deeper and discover what caused your diabetes, you will be cured. That's right, diabetes is 100% reversible, and it can be done 100% without toxic drugs.

You have made a huge step today on the road to be diabetes free.

Take a moment to congratulate yourself on this major life step. Taking a step to head in a healthier direction will have a positive impact on your life and the lives of the people you care about.

Being diagnosed with diabetes can be overwhelming and frightening, but remember this disease process is reversible and something we do every day in our clinic. EVERY DAY patients walk out of our clinic diabetes free.

Unlike most other diabetic books on the market, this book does not tell you what to eat or what medications or supplements to take. Instead, you will learn that diabetes *is a symptom of a deeper-rooted problem.* You'll learn the tools and information to have an intelligent conversation with your physician about digging a little bit deeper into your blood sugar problems.

The unending amount of information can lead anyone to believe reversing diabetes is too difficult and too complicated. In this book, I will cover key concepts proving that it's not – ***once you get to the root of the problem.***

Finally, remember it is important to work with a physician that is well versed in natural medicine such as a naturopathic doctor or functional medicine doctor.

These types of physicians practice what we like to coin as "GET TO THE ROOT OF THE PROBLEM MEDICINE."

So welcome aboard!

CHAPTER 1

THE DIFFERENT TYPES OF DIABETES

We will begin with looking at the different types of diabetes, what are some causes (and there are many!) and what are the differences. When people hear of diabetes, they think of Type 1 and Type 2. There are many other types, and it's important that a diabetic person know which type of diabetes they have. This is because they require different treatment.

Diabetic persons may have:

1. Type 1
2. Type 2
3. Type 1.5; known as Latent Autoimmune Diabetes in Adults (LADA),
4. Type 3 Diabetes

Type 1 Diabetes

5% of the population with diabetes will have type 1. An individual with Type 1 diabetes are often born with it and generally will have had it their entire lives. In type 1 diabetes, the pancreas does not produce enough insulin to effectively regulate blood glucose. So, essentially it is the lack of insulin that is the problem. Treatment available is insulin injections.

For type 1 diabetic patients, the immune system destroys cells in the pancreas. As these cells are destroyed, they can no longer pump out the insulin necessary for lowering blood glucose levels.

While genetics play a role in diabetes development, there are other possible causes. Environmental toxins, viral infections, and hormones can all also play a role.

Type 2 Diabetes

Type 2 is the most common type of diabetes. Type 2 diabetics do produce enough insulin in their pancreas, but the cells of their body do not respond to the insulin. The medical term for this is "insulin resistance."

Insulin is the "key" to unlocking the cell "doors" and allowing glucose into your cells to produce energy. This is how your body produces ENERGY. So, the key (insulin) is not unlocking the door (cell receptor), thus the poor cell has no energy. Your cells then scream to your brain that they are not getting energy and ask the pancreas to release more insulin.

Your pancreas then gets confused thinking it needs to make more insulin and it does. Eventually, the pancreas gets exhausted and start to destroy overworked insulin creating cells called Beta Cells.

A type 2 diabetic may have to start taking additional insulin if too many pancreas cells have been destroyed.

What Causes Type 2 Diabetes?

Weight is a contributor, and people who are overweight tend to develop *insulin resistance* which leads to diabetes.

Toxicity in our environment are big contributors to diabetes. We are bombarded by toxins such as pesticides, herbicides, and heavy metals. Many of these chemicals are known to be hormone disruptors. A big contributor to obesity is a classification of chemicals called "obesegens."

Liver problems could also be a cause for diabetes. The liver is responsible for releasing and storing sugar as your body needs. A dysfunctional liver could be placing unnecessary sugar in your blood stream when it should be storing it.

Other underlying factors that can cause blood sugar problems are:

- Adrenal gland problems
- Thyroid gland problems
- GI imbalances
- Subclinical infections
- Hormone imbalances
- Food sensitivities/allergies

What is Insulin Resistance??

Insulin is a hormone produced by the pancreas that acts to unlock the body's cells so that the glucose (sugar) from the foods we eat can be used by the cells to produce energy. You can think of insulin as the "key" that unlocks the doors (receptor) to your cells. It is vital to get the glucose inside the cell to produce ATP or energy. This is how the human body produces energy.

IMPORTANCE OF INSULIN

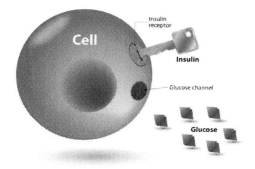

Sometimes the body may not be producing enough insulin to meet their needs, and the cells do not get enough glucose inside of them as a result. In many cases a person's pancreas may actually be producing more insulin than is necessary, in fact, their pancreas is working overtime to produce more insulin, but the body cells are resistant to the insulin. Basically, the cells despite having plenty of insulin in the bloodstream, do not become unlocked and don't let the glucose in the blood to enter the cells. This phenomenon is known as insulin resistance. You have the key (insulin), but the doors aren't unlocking!

Type 1.5; Latent Autoimmune Diabetes in Adults (LADA)

Latent Autoimmune Diabetes in Adults is typed 1.5 because LADA shows characteristics of both type 1 and type 2 diabetes making a clear diagnosis sometimes difficult.

Majority of the time adults develop Type 2 diabetes and children develop Type 1 diabetes. But in Type LADA you can see the reverse where an adult can develop Type 1 diabetes. This makes diagnosis difficult, and LADA tends to be misdiagnosed. About 10% of the diabetic population have LADA. It is slowly progressing, and patients usually do not need insulin as blood sugar can be regulated with lifestyle and diet changes.

Type 3 Diabetes: Alzheimer's

Alzheimer's Disease is Type 3 Diabetes. Alzheimer's is associated with low levels of insulin in the brain. It's becoming clear that lack of insulin – or insulin resistance in the brain, not only impairs memory and cognition but seems to be implicated in the formation of amyloid plaque. When researchers blocked the path of insulin to rodent's brains, their neurons deteriorated rapidly, and their brains showed all the signs of Alzheimer's.

The incidence of Alzheimer's Disease drastically increases with patients diagnosed with Type 2 Diabetes. Women with diabetes have a 137% increase and men with diabetes have a 227% increase. For diabetics that use insulin, there is a *430% chance* of developing Alzheimer's!

Dr. Luminita Alexe, ND

Journal of Alzheimer's Disease 51 (2016) 961-977
DOI 10.3233/JAD-150980
IOS Press

Hypothesis

Unraveling Alzheimer's: Making Sense of the Relationship between Diabetes and Alzheimer's Disease[1]

Melissa A. Schilling*
New York University, New York, NY, USA

Handling Associate Editor: Wei Qiao (Wendy) Qiu

Accepted 11 January 2016

Abstract. Numerous studies have documented a strong association between diabetes and Alzheimer's disease (AD). The nature of the relationship, however, has remained a puzzle, in part because of seemingly incongruent findings. For example, some studies have concluded that insulin deficiency is primarily at fault, suggesting that intranasal insulin or inhibiting the insulin-degrading enzyme (IDE) could be beneficial. Other research has concluded that hyperinsulinemia is to blame, which implies that intranasal insulin or the inhibition of IDE would exacerbate the disease. Such antithetical conclusions pose a serious obstacle to making progress on treatments. However, careful integration of multiple strands of research, with attention to the methods used in different studies, makes it possible to disentangle the research on AD. This integration suggests that there is an important relationship between insulin, IDE, and AD that yields multiple pathways to AD depending on the where deficiency or excess in the cycle occurs. I review evidence for each of these pathways here. The results suggest that avoiding excess insulin, and supporting robust IDE levels, could be important ways of preventing and lessening the impact of AD. I also describe what further tests need to be conducted to verify the arguments made in the paper, and their implications for treating AD.

Keywords: Alzheimer's disease, amylin, amyloid beta-peptide, dementia, diabetes mellitus, insulin, insulysin, metalloproteases, neprilysin

Alzheimer's disease (AD) is a devastating, fatal disease that affects an estimated 5.2 million Americans, and 44 million people worldwide. It is a disease that is often harder on the families and caregivers of the patient than on the patient themselves. The direct costs to the US of AD in 2014 were estimated to total $214 billion [1]. Adding in the informal costs (the costs of family members and friends providing

unpaid care to those with dementia) doubles these figures. The bulk of the financial burden of AD is not due to the cost of drugs or doctor's visits; instead, the vast majority (75–84%) of the expenses go to nursing home care, plus formal and informal home care [2]. The drugs currently available for AD (primarily cholinesterase inhibitors and memantine) offer only incremental improvements in symptoms—they do not stop the progression of the disease [3–6]. Analysts estimate that AD will cost $1.5 trillion per year US by 2050 if a more effective treatment is not developed [7].

[1]New York University Working Paper.
*Correspondence to: Melissa A. Schilling, PhD, New York University, 40 West 4th Street, New York, NY 10012, USA. Tel.: +1 212 998 0316; E-mail: mschilling@stern.nyu.edu.

M.A. Schilling / Unraveling Alzheimer's Disease

AD has been a difficult puzzle to solve, in part because of an abundance of seemingly incongruent findings. For example, though many studies have identified a significant association between type 2 diabetes mellitus (T2DM) and AD (see the review provided in Table 1), these studies have often come to different conclusions about the causal mechanism and its implications for treatment. Some studies, for example, have concluded that insulin deficiency is primarily at fault, suggesting that intranasal insulin or inhibiting the insulin-degrading enzyme (IDE) could be beneficial [8–11]. Other research has concluded that hyperinsulinemia is to blame, which implies that

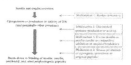

Fig. 1. The insulin-protease-amyloid degradation pathway and its potential malfunctions.

Gestational Diabetes

A woman can develop diabetes when pregnant. This type of diabetes generally occurs only during pregnancy and spontaneously resolves after the baby is born. Hormones within the placenta during pregnancy is responsible for slowing insulin in the mother and worsening insulin resistance.

Gestational diabetes should be monitored very carefully to ensure the health of the mother and baby. Gestational diabetes is serious and could cause serious harm to the mother and baby.

CHAPTER 2

THE RISKS OF TREATING DIABETES WITH DRUGS ARE FAR WORSE THAN THE DISEASE

In 2009, there were nearly 4.6 million drug-related visits to U.S. emergency rooms nationwide, *with more than half* due to adverse reactions to prescription medications. Also in 2009, for the first time ever in the US, more people were killed by prescription drugs than motor vehicle accidents.

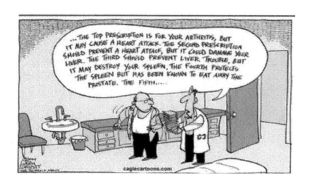

Almost 26 million Americans have diabetes, with over 90% being type 2 diabetes.

Type 1 diabetics is an autoimmune disease and needs insulin injection to keep alive. But type 2 diabetics do NOT need drugs. In fact, diabetes drugs increase your risk of death.

Diabetic drugs are commonly prescribed for type 2 diabetics, but new clinical trials have shown that treatment with glucose-lowering drugs was shown to increase your risk of death.

Researchers noted:

"The overall results of this meta-analysis do not show a benefit of intensive glucose lowering treatment on all-cause mortality or cardiovascular death. A 19% increase in all-cause mortality and a 43% increase in cardiovascular mortality cannot be excluded."

Diabetic Drugs Are Potentially Deadly

Avandia (rosiglitazone), a diabetic drug that hit the market in 1999 was found in a 2007 study to increase the risk of heart attack by 43% and increase cardiovascular death by 64%!

Millions of Americans that have taken Avandia have been exposed to these unacceptable health risks. Over 80,000 diabetics have suffered from heart attacks, strokes or heart failure from this dangerous drug.

It took almost 10 years before the Food and Drug Administration (FDA) took action and restricted access to this drug, while in Europe it was banned altogether.

Avandia is but one example. The New England Journal of Medicine featured not one or two, but FOUR studies stating that conventional medicine is leading diabetics astray and causing more harm than good.

In 2016 the US Food and Drug Administration called attention to the increased risk of amputation if you are on the drug canagliflozin (Invokana, Invokamet). In its statement, the FDA says that:

"Based on new data from two large clinical trials, the FDA has concluded that the type 2 diabetes medicine canagliflozin (Invokana, Invokamet, Invokamet XR) causes an increased risk of leg and foot amputations. FDA requires new warnings, including the most prominent Boxed Warning, to be added to the canagliflozin drug labels to describe this risk."

The risk is about two-fold, the FDA concludes, and most often affects the toe and middle of the foot."

In 2016, the FDA also issued warnings about kidney injury linked with the drug, recommending physicians evaluate kidney health before starting the drug.

This drug primarily works in the kidneys to remove glucose via urine. Unfortunately, I have personally seen this drug do massive damage to many of my patients' kidneys.

Lowering Blood Sugar is Not the Correct Strategy to Overcome Type 2 Diabetes

Diabetes is not a blood sugar disease. Drugs that focus on addressing the *symptom* of high blood sugar are doomed to fail. Drugs treat the symptoms andnot the underlying causes.

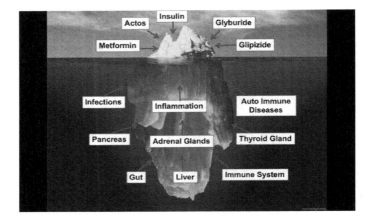

For the last half-century or so, Americans have followed the dietary recommendations of the Food Pyramid which consist of a high complex carbohydrate, low saturated fat diet—the exact *opposite* of what actually works for preventing and reversing diabetes! High complex carbohydrates include legumes, potatoes, corn, rice and grain products. With the exception of legumes, you actually want to AVOID all the rest to prevent insulin resistance and high blood sugar.

"Conventional wisdom" also tells diabetics that table sugar is okay, as long as you readjust your insulin to compensate appropriately. But if you have diabetes, you should be limiting or even eliminating sugar from your diet, especially in the form of fructose.

Type 2 diabetes can be caused by insulin resistance, faulty leptin signaling (leptin is a hormone produced in your fat cells), liver problems, thyroid problems, hormone problems, adrenal problems, gut infections, immune system problems, and more. Drugs are NOT the solution because they do not resolve the underlying problem.

CHAPTER 3

STRESS AND BLOOD SUGAR

When under stress, the body prepares itself by making sure enough sugar or energy will be available in the event of flight or fight. In stressful situations adrenaline, glucagon and cortisol can affect blood sugar greatly. Stressful situations can include anything your body perceives as stress whether physical or emotional/mental. This can include emotional stress, serious illness or infection.

During stressful times epinephrine (adrenaline) and glucagon rise which releases more glucose from the liver. When the stress hormone cortisol levels rise, it causes body tissues (muscle and fat) to not respond to insulin. With tissue not responding to insulin, this increases blood glucose. If you have high levels of stress hormones floating around in your body, you will NOT be able to control your blood sugar optimally.

Stress can also be from low blood sugar levels from too much medication or insulin. The low blood sugar induces a rapid release of stress hormones epinephrine, glucagon, and cortisol. After these powerful hormones are released, it may be difficult to control blood sugar. This phenomenon of low blood sugar followed by high blood sugar is called the "rebound" or "Somogyi" reaction.

During times of stress, a person with diabetes may have more difficulty controlling their blood glucose levels. It is imperative to have stress management techniques to help control blood glucose levels. Control your stress levels or your stress levels will control your blood sugars.

CHAPTER 4

"DIABESITY"; OBESOGENS, WEIGHT, AND DIABETES

Obesity and diabetes have risen steadily in the United States over the past recent decades. 35% of adults and 17% of children aged 2-19 are obese. And those numbers are expected to only increase.

Obesity does not just plague the United States, but worldwide we see record obesity rates. In fact, even animals – pets, lab animals and urban rats are experiencing an increase in body weight. It appears that everyone is gaining weight. So, what's going on?

There's a new group of chemicals that appear to sabotage your ability to regulate weight, regulate your appetite and regulate your blood sugar. Obesogens are chemicals that can promote obesity by increasing the number of fat cells, changing the metabolic rate, and altering hormones that control of satiety and appetite.

These hormones disrupting chemicals can increase your fat cells, alter how you burn calories and even alter the way your body perceives and manages hunger.

We blame our weight gain on eating too many fats, sugars and not getting in enough exercise, but science is discovering that chemicals we are exposed to every day in our food, air, and water play a big part of the obesity epidemic.

In 2011 the NIH launched a 3-year effort to fund research exploring the role of environmental chemical exposures in obesity, type 2 diabetes mellitus, and metabolic syndrome and there is a burst of new data in the last 5 years.

How Obesogens Work In The Body.

1) They reprogram your body cells to become fat cells and encourage your body to store fat. Obesogenic chemicals appeared to have activated peroxisome proliferator-activated receptor gamma (PPARγ), the master regulator of adipogenesis, the process of creating adipocytes, or fat cells.

2) Prevent an appetite reducing hormone called Leptin from being released from your fat cells. This is important because Leptin signals to your body that you are full.

3) Promotes insulin resistance which makes the pancreas release more insulin that turns energy into more fat in the body.

Where Are Obesogens Found?

- Water bottles, cans, and receipts: Bisphenol-A (BPA), a synthetic estrogen that's used to make plastics hard and in the lining of cans, has been shown to increase insulin resistance in animal studies. BPA has also been shown to increase abdominal fat and glucose intolerance.

- Nonstick pans and microwave popcorn: Perfluorooctanoic acid (PFOA), a potential endocrine disruptor and known PPAR γ agonist. It's a widespread chemical, and pretty much everyone in the U.S. has it in their blood. This chemical used to make items non-stick has been shown to lead to obesity and altered Leptin levels which dysregulated metabolism and appetite in animal. It can also affect the thyroid gland, which importantly regulates weight and metabolism. This chemical is found in Teflon coated pans, carpets, pizza boxes, and microwave popcorn bags.

- Air fresheners and shower curtains: Phthalates, are chemicals that are found in fragrance products such as air fresheners and vinyl products such as shower curtains, vinyl flooring, and plastic wrap. Phthalates have been shown to lower metabolism and testosterone, causing you to lose muscle mass and increase fat. Phthalates also increased waist circumference and insulin resistance in adult U.S. males.

- Water: Many chemical pesticides find its way into your tap water. Atrazine is an herbicide and the main obesogen in tap water and has been found to cause mitochondrial dysfunction and insulin resistance. This pesticide was banned in Europe, but not in the United States. Atrazine affects your thyroid by slowing down thyroid hormone metabolism. Tributyltin (TBT), a wood preservative and a fungicide painted on the bottom of boats, is considered an obesogen as has been shown to stimulate fat cell production.

Male mice exposed to low doses of TBT for 45 days show excess weight gain, high insulin levels, and fatty liver. These findings suggest that TBT exposure may lead to obesity, insulin resistance, and fatty liver disease even at very low doses.

Mice chronically exposed to TBT had pancreatic beta cell death, lower insulin levels, and high blood glucose levels

How to Avoid Obesogens.

- Use glass, steel or aluminum water bottles. If you must get plastic, make sure it states that it's a BPA free plastic bottles.
- Get rid of your Teflon or non-stick pans. Opt for ceramic or steel pans to cook in.
- Eliminate chemical air fresheners and opt for natural essential oils instead.
- Eat fewer foods out of a can. Opt for fresh or frozen instead. Some manufacturers now offer BPA free cans.
- Eat meat and milk products that are hormone and antibiotic free. Keep in mind that chemicals concentrate much more on animal products than a plant. Buy wild caught fish instead of farm raised.
- Install water filters on your faucet to filter out chemicals such as atrazine.

CHAPTER 5

DIABETES AND YOUR GUT

If you've been diagnosed with Type 2 diabetes or prediabetes, your doctor has likely told you to focus on healthy eating and exercise to help reduce blood sugar. While good advice, there's increasing evidence that your gut microbiome greatly affects blood sugar. Gut bacteria may play one piece of a very large and complicated puzzle on diabetes.

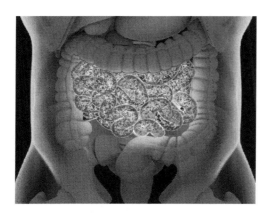

Your gut microbiome is a collection of bacteria in your gastrointestinal tract (GI) that impacts your metabolism, your immunity, synthesizing essential vitamins and amino acids and your ability to extract energy (calories) from food.

Bacteria generate proteins, including hormones, neurotransmitters, and inflammatory molecules, that can enter your blood circulation and affect health. Is it reasonable to assume this can probably affect many major diseases including diabetes and obesity?

The Little Bugs that Directly Cause Obesity.

How do bacteria in the gut affect obesity? First, bacteria influence the calories absorbed by the foods that you eat. Your body weight is not affected by the calories you ingest as much as the calories that are absorbed. Gut bacteria appears to play a huge role in how you're absorbing your calories from the foods you eat. 90% of human gut bacteria will be either Bacteroidetes or Firmicutes. Firmicutes extract more calories than Bacteroidetes. Obese humans have far more Firmicutes, as do rodents.

Various clinical trials have shown the powerful effects bacteria have in the development of obesity in mammals. When gut bacteria from obese mice were transplanted into lean mice, the lean mice became obese despite having the same previous caloric intake.

Further, when gut bacteria from lean mice were transplanted to obese mice, the obese mice became lean. These experiments were reproducible consistently suggesting that gut bacteria influence obesity as well as being a cause of it.

Insulin Signaling Disruption From Your Gut Bacteria.

Gut bacteria imbalance increases the risk of developing insulin resistance. Insulin resistance is the metabolic process involved in the development of pre-diabetes, type 2 diabetes, high blood pressure, and heart disease.

In addition, studies in the past ten years have shown that low-grade inflammation plays a central role in the molecular mechanism of insulin resistance in these diseases.

It appears that bacterial endotoxins affect insulin signaling pathways. An increase in the bacteria Firmicutes and a decrease in Bacteroidetes appear to alter intestinal permeability (leaky gut), increasing the absorption of lipopolysaccharide (LPS) and initiates activation of inflammatory pathways. With the activations of these inflammatory pathways, we see an impairment of insulin signaling.

Research published in the journal *Cellular and Molecular Gastroenterology and Hepatology* have found that in humans, developing type 2 diabetes is also correlated with having bacteria that penetrate the mucus lining of the colon. Bacteria that are able to invade upon the epithelium of the gut promotes inflammation that drives metabolic diseases, specifically type 2 diabetes.

Things You Can Do for a Healthier Gut.

-Adopt a plant-based diet will help improve gut health as plant and fiber-rich diets appear to provide a healthier mix of bacteria.

-Increase probiotic foods such as yogurt, kefir, raw sauerkraut, kimchi, and kombucha. You can also incorporate prebiotics – foods that feed beneficial bacteria. Good sources of prebiotics are garlic, onions, asparagus, leeks, jicama and raw apple cider vinegar.

-Avoid taking unnecessary courses of antibiotics, which greatly disrupts bacteria balance in your gut.

-Find a practitioner that will prescribe probiotic *spores* for you. Unfortunately, most probiotics do not survive the harsh acidic environment of the stomach. Spore probiotics are much more powerful than regular probiotics and have a 100% delivery to the targeted area: your intestines.

CHAPTER 6

10 REASONS FOR BLOOD SUGAR SWINGS

1) **Bad Cold:** Your body can raise your blood sugar to fight infection. Keep in mind that some medicines such as painkillers, antibiotics, and decongestants to clear your sinuses can possibly raise your blood sugar.

2) **Birth Control Pills:** OCP's (Oral Contraceptive Pills) that have estrogen effects the way your body handles insulin.

3) **Caffeine:** Coffee, black tea, green tea, and energy drinks can all raise your blood sugar. Caffeine can elevate cortisol which increases blood sugar levels. It is important to keep track

of your blood sugar response to caffeinated beverages.

4) **Exercise:**   We know that physical activity usually lowers blood sugar because it decreases how much insulin is needed to move sugar into the cells. So, activity lowers blood sugar – but not always! Exercise can trigger the body to release stress hormones such as adrenaline which makes your liver release glucose or cortisol which makes you insulin resistant. There is a small segment of diabetics that have a spike in blood sugar after they exercise.

5) **Stress:**   Unhappy at work or feeling overwhelmed. When under stress your body releases hormones that can make your blood glucose rise. Learn stress relaxation techniques such as deep breathing, journaling or yoga.

6) **Dried Fruit:** Dried versions of fruit will pack more carbohydrate in a smaller serving size. If you must choose, choose fresh fruit over dried.

7) **Sugar-Free Foods:** Although they don't have sugar added, they can still have plenty of carbs from starches. Also, pay attention to sugar alcohols such as xylitol and sorbitol as they have also been known to increase blood sugar levels.

8) **Corticosteroids:** Corticosteroids such as prednisone, used to treat arthritis, asthma, rashes and many other conditions can boost your blood sugar and can even directly trigger diabetes.

9) **Blood Pressure Meds:** Diuretics that are used to treat high blood pressure can also do the same. Certain antidepressants can also raise blood sugar levels.

10) **Cold Medicine:** Pseudoephedrine or phenylephrine found in decongestants can raise blood sugar. Some of these formulas can directly have sugar in them also. Read the labels.

CHAPTER 7:

NATURAL SUPPLEMENTS THAT INCREASE YOUR BLOOD SUGAR

We all hear of supplements that may help lower blood sugar, but what about supplements that may higher your blood sugar? Many natural supplements can affect your blood glucose including melatonin, fish oil, and vitamin C. Just because it is natural does not mean it is safe for YOU. Check with your medical provider before starting any supplements.

Caffeine: Caffeine is found in coffee and teas, energy supplements and drinks and raises blood sugar.

DHEA: DHEA is used for treating many conditions such as aging skin, erectile dysfunction, osteoporosis, and lupus. DHEA can raise blood sugar levels and increase insulin resistance.

Fish Oil: fish oil is used to reduce heart attack risk; however high doses can increase blood sugar levels.

Ginkgo: Ginkgo is used to treat memory impairment, dementia, diabetic retinopathy, and peripheral vascular disease. Ginkgo has been shown to alter insulin secretion and metabolism. It may increase insulin breakdown by the liver, leading to decreased insulin levels and higher blood sugar.

Glucosamine Sulfate: Used to treat joint problems. Glucosamine can increase your blood glucose levels.

Melatonin: Melatonin is a hormone used to treat insomnia and other sleep disorders. It appears to decrease glucose uptake into cells and increases insulin resistance, thus elevating blood sugar. Melatonin can also worsen blood pressure.

Niacin: Niacin and niacinamide, or vitamin B3 are used to lower cholesterol and triglycerides. This vitamin can cause high blood glucose, abnormal glucose tolerance, and glycosuria (sugar loss in urine).

Vitamin C: High doses of vitamin C intake has been shown to increase blood sugar levels.

CHAPTER 8

DIABETIC DIET NO-NO'S

Type 2 diabetes is a disease that is influenced by a lifetime of bad eating habits. It also tends to be accompanied by high cholesterol and high blood pressure. The following foods are big-time sugar disruptors.

Fruit Juice.

Fruit juice contains at least as much sugar as sodas do. Its high fructose content can worsen insulin resistance, promote weight gain and increase the risk of heart disease.

Fruit juice is often considered a healthy drink, but its effects on blood sugar are no different than those of sodas and other sugary drinks.

Fruit juice is loaded with a type of sugar called fructose; this sugar has been proven that it drives insulin resistance, heart disease, and obesity.

A much better alternative is to enjoy flavored seltzer waters as an option or water with a wedge of lemon, which is virtually carb and calorie-free.

Trans Fats.

Trans Fats are a health killer.

They are created by adding hydrogen to unsaturated fatty acids to make them more stable. You may see them labeled as hydrogenated oil or partially hydrogenated oil.

Trans fats are found in crackers, cookies, baked goods, margarines, peanut butter, spreads, creamers and frozen dinners. Trans fats help extend shelf life.

While trans fats won't directly raise blood sugar levels, they are linked to increased insulin resistance and belly fat, as well as lower "good" cholesterol.

This is especially concerning for people with diabetics, as they are at an increased risk of heart attack and stroke.

Trans fats have been outlawed in most countries, and in the US, manufacturers must limit it to .05g per serving.

Until trans fats are no longer in our foods, read the labels and avoid any product that contains the words" hydrogenated" or "partially hydrogenated" in its ingredient list.

White Bread, Pasta, and Rice.

White bread, rice, and pasta are high-carb, processed foods with very little nutrient value.

Consuming bread, bagels and other refined-flour foods has shown to significantly increase blood sugar levels in people with type 1 and type 2 diabetes.

And this increase in blood sugar isn't exclusive to wheat products. Gluten-free breads and pastas were also shown to raise blood sugar, with rice-based types having the greatest effect.

One study found that a meal containing a high-carb bagel not only raised blood sugar but also impaired brain function in people with type 2 diabetes.

White bread, pasta, and rice also contain little fiber, which helps slow down the absorption of sugar into the bloodstream.

Replacing white bread with high-fiber bread was shown to significantly reduce blood sugar levels in people with diabetes.

Remember foods that are high in carbs yet low in fiber are diabetic disasters. This combination will result in high blood sugar levels. Choosing high-fiber, fresh, whole foods may help reduce blood sugar response.

Honey, Agave Nectar, and Maple Syrup.

People with diabetes often try to minimize their intake of white table sugar, as well as treats like candy, cookies, and pie.

However, other natural sugars can also cause blood sugar spikes. These include brown sugar and "natural" sugars like maple syrup, honey, and agave nectar.

Although these sweeteners are more natural; they contain at least as many carbs as white sugar. In fact, most contain *even more.*

Here are the carb counts of a one-tablespoon serving of popular sweeteners:

- **White sugar:** 12.6 grams
- **Agave nectar:** 16 grams
- **Honey:** 17 grams
- **Maple syrup:** 13 grams

People with diabetes and prediabetes experienced similar increases in blood sugar, insulin, and inflammatory markers regardless of whether they consumed 1.7 ounces (50 grams) of white sugar or honey.

Your best strategy is to avoid all forms of sugar and opt for low carb natural sweeteners instead such as Stevia.

Honey, agave nectar and maple syrup appear as a healthier alternative table sugar because they are "natural," but they may have similar effects on blood sugar, insulin, and inflammatory markers.

Dried Fruit.

Fresh fruit is a great source of important vitamins and minerals, including vitamin C, magnesium, and potassium.

When fruit is dehydrated, the process results in a loss of water that leads to even higher concentrations of the sugars in the fruit.

Let's get an example: one cup of grapes contains 27 grams of carbs. By contrast, one cup of raisins contains 115 grams of carbs.

Raisins contain more than three times as much sugar as grapes do. Other types of dried fruit are similarly higher in sugar when compared to fresh fruit.

If you have diabetes, you don't have to give up fruit entirely, but stay away from dehydrated fruit snacks as they pack quite a sugar punch. Low-sugar fruits like fresh berries can keep your blood sugar in the target range while providing health benefits.

Processed Meat.

Conventionally raised red meat and pork (pork is not "the other white meat"), especially processed red meats like sausage, bacon, and hot dogs appear to increase a person's risk of developing type 2 diabetes. The more processed or unprocessed red meat a person eats, the greater the risk, according to a study in the *American Journal of Clinical Nutrition.*

Participants in the study who ate one 3.5-ounce serving of non-processed red meat a day, such as steak or hamburger, were almost 20% more likely to develop type 2 diabetes.

Participants who ate half of this amount of processed meat, such as two slices of bacon or one hot dog, had a 51% increased risk of developing diabetes

It is unknown exactly how red and processed meat affects diabetes. The high amount of nitrate preservatives in processed meat may increase the risk of insulin resistance. Insulin resistance a pre-diabetes occurs when the cells of the body become resistant to the effects of insulin, and glucose cannot enter the cell.

Red meats also contain high amounts of iron and are pro-inflammatory. High total body iron stores have been associated with an elevated risk of type 2 diabetes, according to the study researchers.

Minimize the consumption of processed meat as much as possible and reduce our consumption of conventional red meat and pork. Try to buy organic or antibiotic free and hormone free animal products.

CHAPTER 9

10 DIABETIC SUPERFOODS

1) Asparagus

Diabetic Benefits: Asparagus helps to regulate blood glucose and stimulate the production of insulin.

Cooking: Asparagus can be steamed, broiled or grilled to perfection. Try placing asparagus under fish, wrap in foil and bake in the oven. Both are powerful diabetic foods and delicious with some lemon and seasonings!

2) Avocado

Diabetic Benefits: Avocados have heart-healthy fats and proven to increase "good" cholesterol. They keep electrolytes healthy and do not require a lot of insulin to digest.

Cooking: Avocados can be added to almost anything. Add some on top of meals or salads or add to smoothie.

3) Broccoli

Diabetic Benefits: Broccoli contains a substance called sulforaphane which has been shown to repair the damage in blood vessels that diabetes cause.

Cooking: Steaming is the best way to cook broccoli. Never boil broccoli as the nutrients leach out into the water.

4) Beans

Diabetic Benefits: The almighty little bean truly is a power food. Beans have approximately equal protein, fiber and fats making it a very balanced food. Beans help lower cholesterol and risk of heart disease naturally.

Cooking: Beans can be added to almost anything: add them to a stew for slow cooking or on top of salads for extra protein and fiber.

5) Basil

Diabetic Benefits: Basil is full of antioxidants and essential oils. Basil has been shown to restore pancreatic beta cells and increase insulin production.

Cooking: Basil should not be cooked as it destroys many of its aromatic compounds that have the health benefits. Try chopping and adding on top of dishes or salads.

6) Blueberries

Diabetic Benefits: Blueberries have been proven in studies to help increase insulin sensitivity and help lower blood glucose levels.

Cooking: Mix fresh or frozen blueberries in non-sweetened yogurt or smoothie for a healthy snack.

7) Carrots

Diabetic Benefits: Carrots are high in powerful antioxidants and vitamins such as beta-carotene, folate, magnesium. It helps guard against damage to blood vessels in the eyes.

Cooking: Carrots pack the most nutrient punch when cooked as it weakens the cell wall and nutrients release.

8) Chocolate

Diabetic Benefits: Bet you did not think chocolate was on this list! Dark chocolate has been proven to lower blood sugar in diabetics and decrease insulin resistance. Choose 70% or greater.

Cooking: Hot chocolate with some stevia sweetener or a few small pieces can help satisfy a sweet tooth. Dark chocolate can also be used in certain dishes like chicken or beef mole.

9) Garlic

Diabetic Benefits: Garlic has substances in it that can help stimulate the production of insulin while helping regulate blood sugar all throughout the day.

Cooking: Add chopped or crushed garlic to your stews, stir-frys and salads. Almost any meal goes well with garlic.

10) Ginger

Diabetic Benefits: Ginger is a plant that has been used for hundreds of years. Ginger helps lower blood sugar and increase insulin sensitivity. The American

Diabetes Associate gives this herb overwhelming support for diabetes control.

Cooking: Try shredding and sautéing with your meals. Or make into a hot tea by shredding or cubing a teaspoon and adding to hot water.

CHAPTER 10

IN THE END: YOU CAN REVERSE TYPE 2 DIABETES!

Please don't let anyone tell you that type 2 diabetes has no cure - this is simply not true. At our office, we have successfully reversed thousands of diabetic patient's diabetes and got them off their medications. Type 2 diabetes is not terminal; you do not have to live with diabetes forever!

Nearly 100 percent of type 2 diabetics can be successfully treated – eliminating the high risk of developing health complications such as heart attack, stroke, blindness, kidney failure, and amputation. The main thing that will drastically reduce your risk of the disease is figuring out how you got the disease in the first place. Find a fantastic doctor that can help you uncover the "root" of your disease.

This book is part of a mini-series, the future mini-series will cover specifics on diet, lifestyle, and recipes, but for NOW, here are 7 basic tips to get you started:

1. Severely limit or eliminate grains and sugar from your diet, especially sweetened drinks. This is extremely important! Drinking just one sweetened drink a day can raise your diabetes risk by 25 percent compared to drinking one sugary drink per month, so you really need to evaluate your diet and look for hidden sources of sugar. Artificially sweetened food and drinks should be avoided as well.

2. Eliminate toxins. Remember environmental toxins play a huge rule in insulin receptor disruption and blood sugar disruption.

3. Get plenty of omega 3 fats from sources such as cold water fish and nuts.

4. Monitor your fasting insulin level. This is every bit as important as your fasting blood sugar. You'll want your fasting insulin level to be between 2 to 4. The higher your level, the worse your insulin receptor sensitivity is. Have your doctor monitor your insulin levels as well as glucose levels.

5. Get enough sleep every night.

6. Optimize your vitamin D levels. Maintaining your vitamin D levels around 60-80 ng/ml can significantly help control your blood sugar. Just remember to get your levels tested regularly by your doctor to make sure you're staying within the therapeutic range.

7. Manage your stress and stress hormones. Have your doctor check your stress hormone ranges. Address any underlying emotional issues

and/or stress. Non-invasive tools like yoga, journaling and meditation can be extremely helpful in managing blood sugar.

And finally, remember: Don't treat just the tip of the iceberg with drug therapy, get to the root of the problem to cure your Diabetes once and for all.

REFERENCES:

1. "American Diabetes Association." American Diabetes Association, http://www.diabetes.org/.

2. Alzheimer's Disease Is Type 3 Diabetes–Evidence Reviewed. Suzanne M. de la Monte, Jack R. Wands J Diabetes Sci Technol. 2008 Nov; 2(6): 1101–1113. Published online 2008 Nov.PMCID: PMC2769828

3. "FDA Orders Stronger Warning About Canagliflozin (Invokana) & Amputation Risk." EndocrineWeb, http://www.endocrineweb.com/news/diabetes/57572-fda-orders-stronger-warning-about-canagliflozin-invokana-amputation-risk

4. Schilling, Melissa A. "Unraveling Alzheimer™s: Making Sense of the Relationship between Diabetes and Alzheimer™s Disease1." Journal of Alzheimer's Disease, vol. 51, no. 4, Dec. 2016, pp. 961–977., doi:10.3233/jad-150980.

5. Raatz, S K, et al. "Consumption of Honey, Sucrose, and High-Fructose Corn Syrup Produces Similar Metabolic Effects in Glucose-Tolerant and -Intolerant Individuals." The Journal of Nutrition., U.S. National Library of Medicine, Oct. 2015, www.ncbi.nlm.nih.gov/pubmed/26338891/.

6. "Sugars, Granulated [Sucrose] Nutrition Facts & Calories." Nutrition Data Know What You

Eat.,

nutritiondata.self.com/facts/sweets/5592/2.

7. Boussageon, Rémy, et al. "Effect of Intensive Glucose Lowering Treatment on All Cause Mortality, Cardiovascular Death, and Microvascular Events in Type 2 Diabetes: Meta-Analysis of Randomised Controlled Trials." The BMJ, British Medical Journal Publishing Group, 26 July 2011, http://www.bmj.com/content/343/bmj.d4169

.

8. Deaths: Preliminary Data for 2009." *Read by QxMD Icon*, http://www.readbyqxmd.com/read/25073815/deaths-preliminary-data-for-2009

9. Komaroff, Anthony L. "The Microbiome and Risk for Obesity and Diabetes." Jama, vol. 317, no. 4, 2017, p. 355., doi:10.1001/jama.2016.20099.

10. Diabetes Linked to Bacteria Invading the Colon, Study Finds." ScienceDaily, ScienceDaily, 30 May 2017, http://www.sciencedaily.com/releases/2017/0 5/170530122341.htm

11. Caricilli, Andrea, and Mario Saad. "The Role of Gut Microbiota on Insulin Resistance." Nutrients, vol. 5, no. 3, Dec. 2013, pp. 829– 851., doi:10.3390/nu5030829.

12. Scheithauer, Torsten P.m., et al. "Causality of small and large intestinal microbiota in weight regulation and insulin resistance." Molecular

Metabolism, vol. 5, no. 9, 2016, pp. 759–770., doi:10.1016/j.molmet.2016.06.002.

13. 20 Reasons for Blood Sugar Swings (No. 11 Might Surprise You!)." WebMD, WebMD, http://www.webmd.com/diabetes/daily-control-17/slideshow-blood-sugar-swings

14. Ann, Denise. "Red Meat, Processed Meat Linked to Diabetes Risk." WebMD, WebMD, 10 Aug. 2011, http://www.webmd.com/diabetes/news/2011 0810/red-meat-processed-meat-linked-to-diabetes-risk#1

15. Ashton, J.J. "Supplements to Lower Blood Sugar." LIVESTRONG.COM, Leaf Group, 14 Aug. 2017,

http://www.livestrong.com/article/370053-supplements-to-lower-blood-sugar/

16. Flegal KM, et al. Prevalence and trends in obesity among US adults, 1999–2008. JAMA. 2010;303(3):235–241. http://dx.doi.org/10.1001/jama.2009.2014 [online 17 Jan 2012] [PubMed]

17. Flegal KM, et al. Prevalence of obesity and trends in the distribution of body mass index among US adults, 1999–2010. JAMA. http://dx.doi.org/10.1001/jama.2012.39 [online 17 Jan 2012]. [PubMed]

18. Ogden CL, et al. Prevalence of obesity and trends in body mass index among US children and adolescents, 1999–2010. JAMA.

http://dx.doi.org/10.1001/jama.2012.40
[online 17 Jan 2012]. [PubMed]

19. Evans, Ronald M. "PPARs and the Complex
    Journey to Obesity." The Keio Journal of
    Medicine, vol. 53, no. 2, 2004, pp. 53–58.,
    doi:10.2302/kjm.53.53.

20. PA-12-185: Role of Environmental Chemical
    Exposures in the Development of Obesity,
    Type 2 Diabetes and Metabolic Syndrome
    (R01)." National Institutes of Health, U.S.
    Department of Health and Human Services,
    grants.nih.gov/grants/guide/pa-files/PA-12-
    185.html

21. Lim, Soo, et al. "Chronic Exposure to the
    Herbicide, Atrazine, Causes Mitochondrial
    Dysfunction and Insulin Resistance." PLoS

ONE, vol. 4, no. 4, 2009,
doi:10.1371/journal.pone.0005186.

22. Zuo, Zhenghong, et al. "Tributyltin Causes
Obesity and Hepatic Steatosis in Male
Mice."Environmental Toxicology, vol. 26, no.
1, 2011, pp. 79–85., doi:10.1002/tox.20531.

23. Stahlhut R, et al. Concentrations of urinary
phthalate metabolites are associated with
increased waist circumference and insulin
resistance in adult U.S. males. Environ Health
Perspect. 2007;115(6):876882.
http://dx.doi.org/10.1289/ehp.9882 [PMC
free article] [PubMed]

24. White, Sally S., et al. "Endocrine Disrupting
Properties of Perfluorooctanoic Acid." The
Journal of Steroid Biochemistry and

Molecular Biology, vol. 127, no. 1-2, 2011, pp. 16–26., doi:10.1016/j.jsbmb.2011.03.011.

25. Pu, Yong, et al. "Sex-Specific Modulation of Fetal Adipogenesis by Gestational Bisphenol A and Bisphenol S Exposure." Endocrinology, vol. 158, no. 11, 2017, pp. 3844–3858., doi:10.1210/en.2017-00615.

26. Anari, Razieh, et al. "Sugar-Sweetened Beverages Consumption Is Associated with Abdominal Obesity Risk in *Diabetic Patients.*" *Diabetes & Metabolic Syndrome: Clinical Research & Reviews*, vol. 11, 2017, doi:10.1016/j.dsx.2017.04.024.

Made in the USA
San Bernardino, CA
23 March 2018